ICS 11.020

SCM

世界中医药学会联合会
World Federation of Chinese Medicine Societies

SCM 53—2020

中药处方、调剂、给付与煎服要求 第2部分：中药调剂要求

Requirements for Prescription, Dispensing, Delivery, Decocting and Taking of Chinese Medicine
Part 2: Requirements for Dispensing of Chinese Medicine

世界中联国际组织标准
International Standard of WFCMS

2020-7-2发布实施
Issued & implemented on July 2, 2020

中医古籍出版社
Publishing House of Ancient Chinese Medical Books

图书在版编目（CIP）数据

中药处方、调剂、给付与煎服要求．第2部分，中药调剂要求：汉英对照 / 世界中医药学会联合会著．—北京：中医古籍出版社，2024.5

ISBN 978-7-5152-2453-4

Ⅰ．①中… Ⅱ．①世… Ⅲ．①中药制剂学–汉、英 Ⅳ．① R28

中国版本图书馆 CIP 数据核字（2022）第 011864 号

中药处方、调剂、给付与煎服要求　第2部分：中药调剂要求

世界中医药学会联合会　著

责任编辑　张　楚
封面设计　艺点锦秀
出版发行　中医古籍出版社
社　　址　北京市东城区东直门内南小街16号（100700）
电　　话　010-64089446（总编室）　010-64002949（发行部）
网　　址　www.zhongyiguji.com.cn
印　　刷　北京市泰锐印刷有限责任公司
开　　本　880mm×1230mm　1/16
印　　张　1.75
字　　数　61千字
版　　次　2024年5月第1版　2024年5月第1次印刷
书　　号　ISBN 978-7-5152-2453-4
定　　价　36.00元

目　　次
Contents

前　　言

请注意本文件的某些内容可能涉及专利。本文件的发布机构不承担识别专利的责任。

本文件《中药处方、调剂、给付与煎服要求》分为 4 个部分：

——第 1 部分：中药处方要求；

——第 2 部分：中药调剂要求；

——第 3 部分：中药给付要求；

——第 4 部分：中药煎服要求。

本部分为第 2 部分：中药调剂要求。

主要起草单位：江西中医药大学、加拿大中医药学院、江西省中医药管理局、深圳市卫生健康发展研究和数据管理中心、深圳技术大学、香港浸会大学、澳门科技大学、深圳市卫生健康委员会、深圳市中医院、深圳市标准技术研究院、纽约中医学院、深圳市人民医院、深圳统标科技有限公司、中国人民解放军总医院第五医学中心、中国食品药品检定研究院中药民族药检定所、美国杏林健康科技有限公司、北京中医药大学东方医院、中国中药控股有限公司、澳洲全国中医药针灸学会联合会、澳大利亚澳华中医学会、深圳市中医药企业标准联盟。

参与起草单位：北京中医药大学深圳医院（龙岗）、安徽广印堂中药股份有限公司、澳大利亚中医药学会、北京中医药大学东直门医院、广东食品药品职业学院、亳州市永刚饮片厂有限公司、汕头市澄海区中医医院、德国汉堡大学汉萨美安中医中心、广州市黄埔区穗东街夏园社区卫生服务站、广州市健桥惠泽有限公司、韩国庆熙大学、江西江中中药饮片有限公司、江西省药品检验检测研究院、加州中医药大学、美国金禾中医药有限公司、南方医科大学深圳医院、汕头大学医学院第二附属医院、汕头市澄海区人民医院、汕头市澄海区溪南镇卫生院、汕头市中心医院、汕头市中医医院、上海中医药大学、深圳市华辉药业有限公司、深圳市罗湖区中医院、深圳市药品检验研究院、深圳市中医药学会、首都医科大学附属北京地坛医院、苏州信亨自动化科技有限公司、中国中医科学院中医药信息研究所、中山市中医院。

主要起草人：廖利平、杨明、袁晓宁（加拿大）、肖小河、兰青山、李顺民、曾庆明、吴培凯、邓雪枝、赵永红、陈业孟（美国）、徐子渠、马双成、陈明人、左铮云、朱卫丰、周华、易炳学、李锦轩、林子强（澳大利亚）、杨具荣、姚克勤、程晗、朱丽华、张翼（澳大利亚）、张力、梁晖宙（美国）。

本文件参与起草人及审阅专家（按姓氏拼音排序）：蔡本辉、蔡楚喜、蔡沛彪、蔡文伟、蔡晓纯、蔡永江、陈健星、陈洁、陈镍、陈权韩、谌瑞林、陈思远、陈玩珊、程仕萍、丛佳林、崔欣羽、丁演龄、杜建强、高广印、高新颜、龚千锋、古旭明、关志宇、郭晓秋、何杜朋、何浪、胡世平、胡小婕、胡新华、华国栋、黄剑帆、黄举凯、黄展辉、简晖、赖满香、李静、李锐键、李咏、林韩、林明欣、林树旭、刘宝河、刘炽京（澳大利亚）、刘荣华、刘希伟、刘勇、路海英、罗光明、穆风杨、彭映梅、史花兰、王伽伯、王淑红、王伟群、王越、肖雪青、许素文、许晓瑜、许妍、薛春苗、Yang Woongmo（韩国）、杨西晓、杨晓晖、杨银芳、叶年华、余沐珍、余亚薇、原文鹏、Ron Zaidman（美国）、曾长龙、查青林、章德林、张金莲、张萍、张寿文、章文春、赵恒伯、赵文静、赵振萍（美国）、邹健生。

本文件的起草程序遵守了世界中医药学会联合会发布的《世界中医药学会联合会国际组织标准管理办法》和 SCM 0001–2009《标准制定和发布工作规范》。

引　言

中医药是中华民族的文化瑰宝。中医诊疗服务过程，从病人就诊开始，到医生辨证论治，开具正确的中药处方，再到中药的调剂，各个环节中均有相应关键节点：中医师如何在辨证论治的指导下遣方用药；药房和中药处方如何管理；药事人员如何合规地审方，如何正确地调剂，即中药饮片的给付 / 配方；患者如何自行选购合格的中药饮片进行准确配方和合理煎煮；病人又如何正确服用中药。以上的每一个环节和流程，呈现分散状态，没有形成有机结合，影响中药用药安全与有效，损害消费者切身权益，进而降低中医药服务质量和声誉。

因此，有必要将分散的中药服务环节和流程整合成为一个完整的体系，以标准的形式固化下来，构建一个质量可以追溯的中药服务流程，进而达到减少医疗差错，改善医患关系，避免医疗事故，提高医疗服务水平，保障人民用药安全与有效，维护消费者合法权益的目的。

《中药处方、调剂、给付与煎服要求》旨在整合中医药服务流程，建立、健全中医药标准服务体系与认证制度，规范行业行为和药事人员职业操守，营造中药种植、生产、流通、用药的安全与有效，促进中药贸易公平、公正、和谐和科学发展的良好氛围，让世界各国人民共享中医药发展成果，为全人类的健康作出应有的贡献。

本文件为《中药处方、调剂、给付与煎服要求》第 2 部分，将传统的中药饮片调剂流程分为审方和配方两个部分，其中中药审方部分着重于对中药处方进行审查的过程，审查中药处方格式及书写要求，以“三查七对”为着力点。它与第 1、3、4 部分形成无缝对接，遵循医生辨证论治、理法方药的要求，将中医药的特色和优势传承下来，并且落实到实际工作的操作流程中，以减少调剂、遣方用药的差错，确保用药安全与有效。

中药处方、调剂、给付与煎服要求
第 2 部分：中药调剂要求

1 范围

本文件规定了中药调剂人员的资格要求、调剂室的布局和设施、中药饮片斗谱编排、调剂操作流程以及特殊中药饮片的调剂管理等内容。

本文件适用于医疗机构和药品零售企业对中药的调剂服务。

2 规范性引用文件

下列文件中的内容通过文中的规范性引用而构成本文件必不可少的条款。其中，注日期的引用文件，仅该日期对应的版本适用于本文件；不注日期的引用文件，其最新版本（包括所有的修改单）适用于本文件。

GB/T 7027 信息分类和编码的基本原则与方法

GB/T 7635.1 全国主要产品分类与代码　第 1 部分：可运输产品

GB 12904 商品条码　零售商品编码与条码表示

GB/T 17710 信息技术　安全技术　校验字符系统

GB/T 31773:2015 中药方剂编码规则及编码

GB/T 31774:2015 中药编码规则及编码

GB/T 31775:2015 中药在供应链管理中的编码与表示

SZJG 37.1–2011 中药处方与中药调剂规范　第 1 部分：中药处方

ISO 18662–1 *Traditional Chinese Medicine—Vocabulary—Part 1: Chinese Materia Medica*

ISO 18662–2 *Traditional Chinese Medicine—Vocabulary—Part 2: Processing of Chinese Materia Medica*

ISO 18668–1:2016 *Coding System for Chinese Medicines—Part 1: Coding Rules for Chinese Medicines*

ISO 18668–2:2017 *Coding System for Chinese Medicines—Part 2: Codes for Decoction Pieces*

ISO 18668–3:2017 *Coding System for Chinese Medicines—Part 3: Codes for Chinese Materia Medica*

ISO 18668–4:2017 *Coding System for Chinese Medicines—Part 4: Codes for Granule Forms of Individual Medicinals for Prescriptions*

ISO 20333:2017 *Coding Rules for Chinese Medicines in Supply Chain Management*

ISO 20334:2018 *Coding System of Formulae*

3 术语和定义

下列术语和定义适用于本文件。

3.1
中药饮片

中药材经过炮制后，直接用于中医临床或制剂生产的处方药品。
［来源：ISO 18668–1: 2016，定义 3.3］

3.2
中药调剂

根据中药处方要求，将中药饮片调剂成可供患者使用的剂型的过程。

3.3
中药配方颗粒

由单味中药饮片按传统标准炮制后经提取浓缩制成的、供中医临床配方用的颗粒。又称为单味中药浓缩颗粒剂，商品名及民间称呼还有免煎中药饮片、新饮片、精制饮片、饮料型饮片、科学中药等。

3.4
三查七对

操作前查、操作中查、操作后查，查对床号、查对姓名、查对药名、查对剂量、查对时间、查对浓度、查对用法。

注 1：三查七对就是要提醒医务人员在工作中认真核对，是护理工作的主要制度。延伸为中药的三查七对。

注 2：中药的三查七对。三查：一查，医生是否获得当地卫生行政部门或行业管理部门认可的处方权，有开具处方资质；二查，处方书写格式和要求，是否符合当地卫生行政部门和行业管理部门政策法规的要求；三查，中药处方质量，医生辨证论治、理法方药、配伍禁忌（十八反、十九畏，妊娠用药），以及《麻醉药品和精神药品管理条例》等有关文件。七对：一对，一般项目，包括医疗机构名称、费别、患者姓名、性别、年龄、门诊或住院病历号、科别或病区床位号等；二对，辨证论治，中医诊断，包括病名和证候，医嘱；三对，理法方药，药品名称、用量、用法，中成药还应标明剂型、规格；剂量使用公制单位，用阿拉伯数字书写，一般应以克（g）为单位；四对，检查处方的“君、臣、佐、使”的顺序排列；五对，对中药饮片的规格，生用或者制用，配伍禁忌，十八反、十九畏；六对，医师签名或加盖专用签章、处方日期；七对，药品金额，审核、调配、核对、发药药师签名或者加盖专用签章。

3.5
理法方药

中医辨证论治完整体系的高度概括。理法是遣方用药的依据，方药是明理立法的体现。由于病人患病有外感内伤之别，病症表现有寒热虚实之分，兼之年龄、体质、方土、习俗等方面的个体差异，决定了中医组方用药，既有一定法度，又应灵活权变。

3.6
医疗用毒性药品

根据各国家和地区要求，列入“医疗用毒性药品目录”的药品。

注：医疗用毒性药品简称毒性药品。

4 调剂人员资格要求

4.1 调剂人员的资质应符合当地卫生、行业管理的要求。

4.2 调剂人员签名或者专用签章式样应在本机构留样备查。

4.3 调剂人员应每年至少体检一次。凡患有精神疾病及可能影响药品质量的传染病、皮肤病的调剂人员，在未治愈前，都不得参加中药调剂工作。

5 调剂室布局与设施

5.1 布局要求

调剂室布局应满足工作需要，符合中药房基本设施相关要求。

5.2 设施要求

5.2.1 中药调剂室应有足够的面积和空间，室内墙面、地面、顶棚应光滑、无缝隙，不应有颗粒性物质脱落。墙面宜采用防水、防潮、防霉装修材料，可耐受擦洗。有空气调温、调湿等设施，有防潮、防霉、防火、防鼠、防水、防盗、遮阳等设施。

5.2.2 中药饮片调剂设备（器具）主要包括：药斗（架）、调剂台、称量用具（药戥、电子秤等）、粉碎用具（铜缸或小型粉碎机）、冷藏柜、新风除尘设备（可根据实际情况选配）、贵重药品柜、毒麻药品柜。

6 中药饮片斗谱编排

6.1 斗谱编排原则

斗谱编排应满足以下要求：

——有利于减轻劳动强度，方便调剂和加药。

——有利于避免发生差错事故。

——有利于记忆。

——有利于中药饮片管理。

——有利于人员分工合作。

6.2 屉斗标签

标签上应使用中药饮片标准名称。

7 调剂操作规程

7.1 审方

7.1.1 调剂人员在接到中药处方时，应进行三查七对。查处方，核对科别、姓名、年龄。核对药品，需核对药名、剂型、规格、数量等内容。

7.1.2 核查配伍禁忌、妊娠禁忌、医疗用毒性中药、含罂粟壳处方，配伍禁忌药和妊娠禁忌药参见附录 A 表 A.1 和表 A.2。

7.1.3 核对药品性状、用法用量。核查用药合理性，核对临床诊断。超出处方时效和剂量的应对中药处方进行时效性调配。不规范的处方或者不能判定其合法性的处方，不应调剂。

7.2 调配

7.2.1 根据处方药物的不同体积和重量，选用适当的计量工具。如使用电子秤或天平，每次调配前要清零或调零。

7.2.2 对于一方多剂的处方应按“等量递减”的原则，每一剂的重量误差应控制在 ±5% 以内。

7.2.3 调配时，应注意避免撒药及药斗之间掺混的现象。

7.2.4 为便于核对，要按处方药味所列的顺序调配，间隔平放，不可混放一堆。

7.2.5 按照中医师的处方要求进行调配。调配含有毒性中药饮片的处方，对处方未注明“生用”的，如有炮制品，应给付炮制品。注意不可生制不分，以生代制。

7.2.6 处方中如有鲜药，应洗净泥土，去掉非药用部分，切剪成段单包，以免干湿相混，发霉变质，影响疗效。

7.2.7 处方中有需要特殊处理的药品，如先煎、后下、包煎、冲服、烊化、另煎等，要单包成小包并注明用法。附录 A 表 A.3 给出了常见需要特殊处理的药品。

7.2.8 矿物类、动物贝壳类、果实种子类等质地坚硬的药品，需要临时捣碎后再分剂量，以利于煎出有效成分。附录 A 表 A.4 给出了需临时捣碎的常用中药饮片。

7.2.9 处方中有需要临时炮制加工的药品应按照相关规范，依法进行炮制。

7.2.10 小包装中药饮片调剂应遵循相关规定。

7.2.11 急诊处方应先调配，以免延误治疗。

7.2.12 调配完毕，经自查确认无误签名或者加盖专用签章后，再交由复核人员进行复核。

7.3 复核

7.3.1 审查调配好的药品是否与处方所开药味及剂数相符，有无错味、漏味、多味和掺杂异物。

7.3.2 审查称好的药品剂量是否与处方用量有差距，处方中各味药的剂量应准确，每剂药的剂量误差应控制在 ±5% 以内。必要时需重新称量。

7.3.3 审查十八反、十九畏、妊娠禁忌、超过常用剂量等可能引起用药安全的问题，以及毒性中药、麻醉中药、贵细药品的调配是否得当。

7.3.4 审查需先煎、后下、包煎、烊化、另煎、冲服等特殊处理的药品是否单包并注明用法。

7.3.5 审查药品质量，有无虫蛀、发霉变质等。

7.3.6 审查有无乱代乱用等现象，有无生制不分或以生代制，以及应捣未捣等。

7.3.7 住院处方或代煎药，还应复核煎药瓶签与处方上的姓名、科室、送药日期、剂数。

7.3.8 复核人员检查无误后，应签名或者加盖专用签章，方可包装药品。

8 特殊中药饮片调剂管理

特殊中药饮片调剂管理应符合各国家和地区卫生管理部门的相关规定，也可参考附录 A 执行。

附录 A
（资料性）
特殊中药饮片调剂要求

A.1 特殊中药饮片的调剂管理

A.1.1 医疗用毒性中药饮片调剂与管理

毒性中药需设毒剧药柜，实行专人、专账、专柜加锁保管，并贴明标签。

医疗单位供应和调配毒性中药，应凭医生签名的处方。调配处方时，应认真负责，计量准确，按医嘱注明要求，并由配方人员及具有中药师以上技术职称的复核人员签名盖章后方可发出。对处方未注明“生用”的毒性中药，应付炮制品。如发现处方有疑问时，应经原处方医生重新审定后再行调配。

毒性中药应设立专账卡，日清月结，做到账物相符，并填写使用登记本，登记本上应写明患者姓名、年龄、单位、联系方法、使用药品名称、数量及期限，处方医生姓名、调配人员姓名。

处方一次有效，取药后处方及证明保存 2 年备查。

毒性中药管理品种范围及用法用量见 SZJG 37.1–2011《中药处方与中药调剂规范　第 1 部分：中药处方》。

A.1.2 麻醉药品管理中药饮片调剂与管理

中药调剂人员应凭麻醉药品专用处方配药，对不合法、不合理处方，药学部门有权拒绝调配。

调剂麻醉药品处方应专册登记，登记内容包括：处方日期、科别、患者姓名、病历号、性别、年龄、诊断、罂粟壳用量、医师姓名、调剂人、核对人。

处方不得重复取药，取药后需由医疗机构保存 3 年备查。

A.1.3 贵重中药饮片调剂与管理

贵重中药品种见 SZJG 37.1–2011《中药处方与中药调剂规范　第 1 部分：中药处方》。

凡属一类贵重药品，明细收支台账的内容应包括：“日期”“事件摘要”“进、销、存数量”“发药人”“核对人”。发药处方逐张登记，集中存放，在“事件摘要”项下应登记病人姓名和处方号等。

相关管理人员应每日根据门诊用药消耗数量，及时补充药品以保证临床用药，当日消耗的贵重药品应及时登记入账，并应账物相符。

贵重药品应定期检查，严防过期霉变的现象发生，易变质的药品应存放于带锁的冷柜中。

A.2 特殊中药饮片列表

A.2.1 配伍禁忌药

配伍禁忌药见表 A.1。

表 A.1 配伍禁忌药

十八反	甘草反甘遂、大戟、芫花、海藻；乌头（川乌、草乌、附子）反贝母（川贝母、浙贝母、平贝母、伊贝母、湖北贝母）、瓜蒌（瓜蒌、瓜蒌子、瓜蒌皮、天花粉）、半夏、白蔹、白及；藜芦反人参、丹参、沙参、玄参、苦参、细辛、芍药（白芍、赤芍）
十九畏	硫黄畏朴硝，水银畏砒霜，狼毒畏密陀僧，巴豆畏牵牛，丁香畏郁金，川乌、草乌畏犀角，牙硝畏三棱，官桂畏石脂，人参畏五灵脂。

A.2.2 妊娠禁忌药

妊娠禁忌药见表 A.2。

表 A.2 妊娠禁忌药

禁用药	三棱、莪术、水蛭、虻虫、甘遂、京大戟、芫花、牵牛子、巴豆、千金子、商陆、轻粉、斑蝥、雄黄、麝香、猪牙皂、益母草、马钱子、附子、土鳖虫、川牛膝、玄明粉、芒硝、阿魏、闹羊花、蜈蚣等
慎用药	蟾酥、华山参、制天南星、干漆、急性子、硫黄、制川乌、制草乌、白附子、枳实、枳壳、大黄、番泻叶、肉桂、凌霄花、木鳖子、牛膝、红花、桃仁、三七、郁李仁、虎杖、卷柏、王不留行、禹州漏芦、漏芦、片姜黄、西红花、穿山甲、冰片、苏木、通草、常山、蒲黄、赭石、瞿麦等

A.2.3 需要特殊煎煮的中药饮片

需要特殊煎煮的中药饮片见表 A.3。

表 A.3 需要特殊煎煮的中药饮片

先煎	龟甲、鳖甲、赭石、石决明、牡蛎、龙骨、磁石、石膏、紫石英、寒水石、自然铜、蛤壳、珍珠母、鹿角霜、瓦楞子、制川乌、制草乌、制附子、制白附子、商陆、生天南星、生半夏、石斛等
后下	薄荷、砂仁、豆蔻、沉香、苦杏仁、钩藤、大黄、番泻叶、徐长卿、青蒿、鱼腥草等
包煎	葶苈子、车前子、旋覆花、生蒲黄、六一散、黛蛤散、益元散、蛤粉、青黛、马勃、滑石粉、海金沙、儿茶等
冲服	牛黄、三七粉、珍珠、朱砂、麝香、熊胆、马宝、猴枣、羚羊角粉、沉香粉、琥珀粉、玳瑁粉、川贝母、湖北贝母、雷丸等
烊化	阿胶、鹿角胶、龟甲胶、蜂蜜、饴糖等
另煎	人参、天麻、羚羊角片、西洋参、西红花、冬虫夏草、鹿茸片等
溶化	芒硝、玄明粉等

A.2.4 需临时捣碎的常用中药饮片

需临时捣碎的常用中药饮片见表 A.4。

表 A.4 需临时捣碎的常用中药饮片

果实和种子类	丁香、刀豆、大枣、川楝子、五味子、牛蒡子、白果、白扁豆、瓜蒌子、决明子、红豆蔻、豆蔻、芥子、诃子、青果、郁李仁、使君子、胡椒、荜茇、草豆蔻、草果、荔枝核、牵牛子、砂仁、桃仁、莱菔子、益智、预知子、猪牙皂、黑芝麻、榧子、酸枣仁、蔓荆子、蕤仁、橘核等
根和根茎类	山慈菇、平贝母、竹节参、华山参、珠子参、绵马贯众等
矿物类	白矾、自然铜等
动物类	海马、鹿角霜、穿山甲、鳖甲、龟甲等
其他药	儿茶、肉桂等

Foreword

Note that certain contents of this document may involve certain patents. The issuing authority of this document assumes no statutory duty to identify the patent.

The series of standards of *Requirements for Prescription, Dispensing, Delivery, Decocting and Taking of Chinese Medicine* are divided into 4 parts.

- *Part 1: Requirements for Prescription of Chinese Medicine*
- *Part 2: Requirements for Dispensing of Chinese Medicine*
- *Part 3: Requirements for Delivery of Chinese Medicine*
- *Part4: Requirements for Decocting and Taking of Chinese Medicine*

This document is the second part: *Requirements for Dispensing of Chinese Medicine.*

The main drafting organizations: Jiangxi University of Chinese Medicine, College of Traditional Chinese Medicine of Canada, Jiangxi Administration of Traditional Chinese Medicine, Shenzhen Health Development Research and Data Management Center, Shenzhen Technology University, Hong Kong Baptist University, Macau University of Science and Technology, Health Commission of Shenzhen Municipality, Shenzhen Hospital of Traditional Chinese Medicine, Shenzhen Institute of Standards and Technology, NewYork College of Traditional Chinese Medicine, Shenzhen People's Hospital, Shenzhen Unified Standard Technology Co., Ltd., The Fifth Medical Center of the General Hospital of the Chinese People's Liberation Army, Inspection Office of Traditional Chinese Medicine of National Institute for Food and Drug Control, USA Hingli Health and Technology Co., Ltd, Dongfang Hospital of Beijing University of Chinese Medicine, China Traditional Chinese Medicine Holdings Co., Ltd., Federation of Chinese Medicine and Acupuncture Societies of Australia (FCMA), Australian Austro-Central China Medical Association and Shenzhen Standards Alliance for Traditional Chinese Medicine Enterprises.

The drafting organizations participants: Shenzhen Hospital of Beijing University of Chinese Medicine (Longgang), Anhui Guangyintang Traditional Chinese Medicine Co., Ltd., Chinese Medicine & Acupuncture Society of Australia, Dongzhimen Hospital of Beijing University of Chinese Medicine, Guangdong Food and Drug Vocational College, Bozhou Yonggang Decoction Pieces Factory Co., Ltd., Chenghai Hospital of Traditional Chinese Medicine, HanseMerkur Center for Traditional Chinese Medicine at the University Medical Center Hamburg-Eppendorf gGmbH in Germany, Xiayuan Community Health Service Station of Suidong, Huangpu, Guangzhou, Guangzhou Jianqiao Huize Co., Ltd., Korea KyungHee University, Jiangxi Jiangzhong TCM Decotion Pieces Co., Ltd., Jiangxi Institute for Drug Control, Five Branches University of California, USA Kamwo Meridian Herbs, Shenzhen Hospital of Southern Medical University, The Second Affiliated Hospital of Shantou University Medical College, People's Hospital of Chenghai, Shantou, Health Center of Xinan, Chenghai, Shantou, Shantou Central Hospital, Shantou Hospital of Traditional Chinese Medicine, Shanghai University of Traditional Chinese Medicine, Shenzhen Huahui Pharmaceutical Co., Ltd., Shenzhen Luohu District Hospital of Traditional Chinese Medicine, Shenzhen Institute for Drug Control, Shenzhen Society of Traditional Chinese

Medicine, Beijing Ditan Hospital of Capital Medical University, Suzhou Xinheng Automation Technology Co., Ltd, Institute of Information on Traditional Chinese Medicine of China Academy of Chinese Medical Sciences, Zhongshan Hospital of Traditional Chinese Medicine.

The main drafters : Liao Liping, Yang Ming, Yuan Xiaoning (Canada), Xiao Xiaohe, Lan Qingshan, Li Shunmin, Zeng Qingming, Wu Peikai, Deng Xuezhi, Zhao Yonghong, Chen Yemeng (United States), Xu Ziqu, Ma Shuangcheng, Chen Mingren, Zuo Zhengyun, Zhu Weifeng, Zhou Hua, Yi Bingxue, Li Jinxuan, Lin Ziqiang(Australia), Yang Jurong, Yao Keqin, Cheng Han, Zhu Lihua, Kevin Chang (Australia), Zhang Li and Liang Huizhou (United States).

Drafting participants and reviewing experts(in alphabetical order of Surname): Cai Benhui, Cai Chuxi, Cai Peibiao, Cai Wenwei, Cai Xiaochun, Cai Yongjiang, Chen Jianxing, Chen Jie, Chen Nie, Chen Quanhan, Chen Ruilin, Chen Siyuan, Chen Wanshan, Cheng Shiping, Cong Jialin, Cui Xinyu, Ding Yanling, Du Jianqiang, Gao Guangyin, Gao Xinyan, Gong Qianfeng, Gu Xuming, Guan Zhiyu, Guo Xiaoqiu, He Dupeng, He Lang, Hu Shiping, Hu Xiaojie, Hu Xinhua, Hua Guodong, Huang Jianfan, Huang Jukai, Huang Zhanhui, Jian Hui, Lai Manxiang, Li Jing, Li Ruijian, Li Yong, Lin Han, Lin Mingxin, Lin Shuxu, Liu Baohe, Liu Chijing(Australia), Liu Ronghua, Liu Xiwei, Liu Yong, Lu Haiying, Luo Guangming, Mu Fengyang, Peng Yingmei, Ron Zaidman (United States), Shi Hualan, Wang Jiabo, Wang Shuhong, Wang Weiqun, Wang Yue, Xiao Xueqing, Xu Suwen, Xu Xiaoyu, Xu Yan, Xue Chunmiao, Yang Woongmo (South Korea), Yang Xixiao, Yang Xiaohui, Yang Yinfang, Ye Nianhua, Yu Muzhen, Yu Yawei, Yuan Wenpeng, Zeng Changlong, Zha Qinglin, Zhang Delin, Zhang Jinlian, Zhang Ping, Zhang Shouwen, Zhang Wenchun, Zhao Hengbo, Zhao Wenjing, Zhao Zhenping (United States), and Zou Jiansheng.

The drafting procedure of this document complies with the *Standard Management Measures for International Organizations of the World Federation of Chinese Medicine Societies and* SCM 0001–2009 *Standards Development and Publication Work Specification* issued by WFCMS.

Introduction

Traditional Chinese Medicine(TCM) is a cultural treasure of the Chinese nation. The process of TCM diagnosis and treatment starts from the patient's treatment, to the doctor's treatment based on syndrome differentiation, issuing the correct TCM prescription, and then dispensing the decoction pieces, there are corresponding key nodes in each link: How the TCM physician dispenses the prescription under the guidance of treatment based on syndrome differentiation; How to manage pharmacies and TCM prescriptions; How to check the prescription in compliance and how to adjust the prescription correctly, that is the dispensing/delivery of decoction pieces; How patients choose qualified decoction pieces for accurate formulation and reasonable decocting; How patients take Chinese medicine correctly. Each of the above links and processes is scattered without organic integration, which affects the safety and effectiveness of TCM use, damages the vital rights and interests of consumers, and further reduces the quality and reputation of TCM service.

Therefore, it is necessary to integrate the scattered TCM service links and processes into a complete system, solidified in a standard form, and build a TCM service process with traceable system, so as to reduce medical errors, improve the relationship between doctors and patients, avoid medical accidents, improve the level of medical services, ensure the safety and effectiveness of people's medication, and safeguard the legitimate rights and interests of consumers.

The purpose of the series of standards of *Requirements for Prescription, Dispensing, Delivery, Decocting and Taking of Chinese Medicine* is to integrate the service process of TCM, establish and improve the standard service system and certification system of TCM, standardize the industry behavior and the professional ethics of pharmaceutical personnel, create a safe and effective cultivation, production, circulation and drug use of TCM, promote a good atmosphere of fair, just, harmonious and scientific development of TCM trade. What's more important is that people around the world share the fruits of TCM development and make due contribution to the health of mankind.

This document is part 2. Dispensing of Chinese medicines consists of two sections: prescription reviewing and prescription filling. Prescription reviewing mainly focuses on the procedure of prescription checking strictly in accordance with principles of "three reviews and seven checks". This part, which forms a seamless connection with 1, 3 and 4 parts, abiding by syndrome differentiation and treatment as well as requirements of principle-method-recipe-medicines to inherit the characteristics and advantages of TCM, and put them into specific operation processes of medical practice, aiming to reducing mistakes and errors in prescription dispensing and filling, ensuring medication safety and effectiveness, and safeguarding the vital interests of consumers.

Requirements for Prescription, Dispensing, Delivery, Decocting and Taking of Chinese Medicine
Part 2: Requirements for Dispensing of Chinese Medicine

1 Scope

This document specifies the regulations for the qualifications of Chinese medicine dispensing, arrangement and facilities of dispensing rooms, the index of decoction pieces and Chinese patent medicine in the medicine cupboard, the dispensing process, as well as dispensing management for the special medicines.

This document is applicable to carry out Chinese medicine dispensing services of medical institutions and drug retail enterprises.

2 Normative Reference

The following documents are indispensable for the application of this document. As for the dated references, only the dated versions apply to this document. As for the undated references, the latest edition (including all amendments) are applicable to this document.

GB/T 7027 *Basic Principles and Methods for Information Classifying and Coding*

GB/T 7635.1 *National Central Product Classification and Codes—Part 1: Transportable Product*

GB 12904 *Bar Code for Commodity—Retail Commodity Numbering and Bar Code Marking*

GB/T 17710 *Information Technology—Security Technique—Check Character Systems*

GB/T 31773-2015 *Coding Rules for Chinese Medicinal Formulae and their Codes*

GB/T 31774-2015 *Coding Rules for Chinese Medicines and their Codes*

GB/T 31775-2015 *Coding Rules for Chinese Medicines in Supply Chain Management*

SZJG 37.1-2011 *Specification of Prescription and Dispensing of Traditional Chinese Medicine—Part 1: Prescription of Traditional Chinese Medicine*

ISO 18662-1 *Traditional Chinese Medicine—Vocabulary—Part 1: Chinese Materia Medica*

ISO 18662-2 *Traditional Chinese Medicine—Vocabulary—Part 2: Processing of Chinese Materia Medica*

ISO 18668-1:2016 *Coding System for Chinese Medicines—Part 1: Coding Rules for Chinese Medicines*

ISO 18668-2:2017 *Coding System for Chinese Medicines—Part 2: Codes for Decoction Pieces*

ISO 18668-3:2017 *Coding System for Chinese Medicines—Part 3: Codes for Chinese Materia Medica*

ISO 18668-4:2017 *Coding System for Chinese Medicines—Part 4: Codes for Granule forms of*

Individual Medicinals for Prescriptions

ISO 20333:2017 *Coding Rules for Chinese Medicines in Supply Chain Management*

ISO 20334:2018 *Coding System of Formulae*

3 Terms and Definitions

For the purposes of this document, the following terms and definitions apply.

3.1

Decoction Pieces

The processed and prescripted Chinese medicine which are directly used in clinical or pharmacy producing.

[Source ISO 18668-1:2016, definition 3.3]

3.2

Dispensing of Chinese Medicine Decoction Pieces

The process of dispensing the medicine pieces into the suitable dosages for patients' use in accordance with the requirements of Chinese medicine prescription.

3.3

Chinese Medicine Formula Granules

Granules made from single herbal pieces processed according to traditional standards and then extracted and concentrated for the clinical formulation of Chinese medicine, which is also called single Chinese medicine concentrated granules, the trade name and folk name include decoction-free pieces, new pieces, refined pieces, beverage-type pieces, scientific Chinese medicine, etc.

3.4

Three Reviews and Seven Checks

Three reviews refer to prescription reviewing before, during and after of its dispensing. Seven checks refer to check the bed number, check the name, check the drug name, check the dose, check the time, check the concentration, check the usage.

Notes 1: The purpose of three reviews and seven checks is to remind medical staff to check carefully at work, which has always been the major system of nursing work. Extension to Chinese medicine has another meaning.

Notes 2: Three reviews and seven checks in Chinese medicines.Three reviews: First, inquiry into whether the doctor has the prescribing authority recognized by the local health administrative department or industry management department to prescribe; Second, inquiry into whether the prescription writing format and requirements comply with local health and industry management policies and regulations; Third, inquiry into the quality of Chinese medicine prescriptions, the doctor's treatment based on syndrome differentiation, the rationale for prescriptions, the contraindications (eighteen clashes and nineteen incompatibilities, pregnancy medication), and the *Regulations on the Administration of Narcotic Drugs and Psychotropic Substances*, etc. Seven checks: First, general items: including medical institution name, fee, patient name, gender, age, outpatient or inpatient medical record number, department or ward bed number, etc; Second, treatment based on syndrome differentiation, diagnosis, including disease name and syndrome, doctor's advice; Third, priniciple-method-recipe-medicines, and for prescription medicines, the name, dosage and usage of the medicine, the dosage form and specification of the Chinese patent medicine shall also be indicated; the dosage shall be written in metric units and written in Arabic numerals, generally in grams (g); Fourth, check the order of "monarch, minister, assistant, envoy" of the prescription; Fifth, specifications of decoction pieces, for raw or prepared use, incompatibility, eighteen clashes and nineteen incompatibilities; Sixth, physician's signature or special seal, prescription date; Seventh, the amount of the drug, audited, dispensed, checked, signed by the pharmacist issuing the drug or stamped with a special seal.

3.5
Principle-method-recipe-medicines

It is a high-level summary of the complete system of TCM syndrome differentiation and treatment. Method refers to the basis for prescription medication, prescription is the embodiment of using TCM theories. The patient's illness is different from exogenous diseases and internal impairment, the symptoms of the disease are divided into cold and heat, deficiency and excess, and in addition individual differences in age, physique, recipe, customs, etc., it determines the prescription of Chinese medicine and has certain principles and flexibility.

3.6
Toxic Medicine

Medicines listed in the "List of Toxic Drugs for Medical Use" according to the requirements of various countries and regions.

Note: Toxic drugs for medical use are referred to as toxic medicines.

4 Qualifications of Dispensing Stuff

4.1 Qualifications of the dispensing personnel shall meet the requirements of local health, industry management.

4.2 Specimen of the dispensing stuff's signature or special seal shall be submitted to related administrative institution for future reference.

4.3 Dispensing stuff should undertake physical examinations at least once a year. Practitioners suffering from mental disorder or infectious diseases or dermatosis, which might affect medicinal qualification, should not dispense medicines until they have recovered.

5 Arrangement and Facilities for Dispensing Room

5.1 Requirements on the Arrangement

The arrangement of dispensing room should meet the operational requirements and comply with the rules for basic facilities of TCM pharmacy.

5.2 Requirements on the Facilities

5.2.1 There should be adequate area and space in the dispensing rooms, and the walls, floor and ceiling should be smooth and free of cracks. There must be no granular material falling off. The wall should be covered with waterproof, moisture-proof and mildew proof decorating materials, which should also withstand scrubbing. Facilities used for air conditioning, moisture adjustment, moisture-proof, mildew proof, fire prevention, anti-mouse, waterproof, anti-theft, sun shading and others should be installed.

5.2.2 Chinese decoction pieces dispensing devices or equipment mainly include decoction piece drawers or shelfs, dispensing worktop, weighing equipment (including pieces steelyard, electronic scale, etc.), grinding tools (copper herb grander or mini-type crusher), refrigerated cabinets, fresh air and dust removing facilities (if needed), and cabinets for expensive, toxic and anesthetic medicines. Chinese patent medicine dispensing devices or equipment mainly include drug shelves, dispensing worktop, cabinets for expensive medicines and refrigerators.

6 Layout of Decoction Pieces and Classification and Placement of Patent Medicine

6.1 Layout of Decoction Pieces

Decoction pieces layout should meet the following requirements:

— For reducing labor intensity and for the convenience of dispensing and adding decoction pieces.

— For avoiding errors and accidents.

— For the convenience of memorizing each piece's location.

— For decoction pieces management.

— For division of labor and cooperation.

6.2 Chinese Patent Medicine Classification and Placement

Standard names of decoction pieces should be written on the tabs.

7 Dispensing Procedures

7.1 Receiving and Reviewing

7.1.1 When the prescriptions being received, practitioners should check them, including the basic information and make sure the correctness of medical department, patients' name and age. Check the medicines in terms of their names, dosage, specification and quantity.

7.1.2 Checking the compatibility avoidances, pregnancy contradictions, toxic medicines and the prescriptions with Pericarpium Papaveris. Annex A table A.1 and A.2 are for the references of compatibility avoidances and pregnancy contradictions.

7.1.3 Checking the properties, administration and dosage of medicines. Checking the validity of medication and clinical diagnosis. Conduct timeliness deployment on prescription beyond expiration and dosage. Prescriptions below standard or without validity are not allowed to be dispensed.

7.2 Dispensing

7.2.1 Weighting tools should be used according to the size and weight of medicine. Scale or electronic scale should be reset before using.

7.2.2 When one formula is prescribed in multiple dosages, weights of each dosage should be reduced sequentially and gradually, and the weight error should be controlled within ± 5%.

7.2.3 When dispending, practitioners should avoid herbs dropping or mixing-up of decoction pieces between drawers.

7.2.4 In order to make it easier for checking, the herbs should be placed in sequence of the prescription, and lined up in separate piles instead of being mixed.

7.2.5 Doctor's prescription should be followed during dispensing. As for the toxic medicines, if they are not noted unprocessed use, the processed ones should be dispensed. Failing to distinguish the crude medicine from the processed one or replace the processed one with the processed ones should be avoided.

7.2.6 As for the fresh medicines in the prescriptions, the dirt on them should be removed. After which, they should be cut up into pieces and packed separately, rather than store them with dry ones, which may get them rotten and influence the medical effects.

7.2.7 As for the special-dealt medicines, including decocted earlier, decocted later, wrap-boiling, dissolving or melting, decocted separately should be packed into small and separate packages and note the usage. The common special-dealt medicines are listed in Annex A table A.3.

7.2.8 Medicinal of hard texture like minerals, animal shells and seeds are to be dispensed after mashing and crushing, which is helpful to extract the active agents. Common items requiring crush and mash are listed in Annex A table A.4.

7.2.9 Medicines demanding temporary processing should be done as the procedures written accordingly.

7.2.10 Decoction pieces in small package should be dispensed as the procedures written accordingly.

7.2.11 Emergency prescription should be dispensed in advance in order to avoid delaying treatment.

7.2.12 After dispensing and checking, the dispenser should sign their names or seal and send it to the reviewers.

7.3 Reviewing

7.3.1 Recheck the amount and dosages of the dispensing medicine and whether there's any wrong, excessive and foreign matters being mixed in or missing.

7.3.2 Checking whether there is a gap between the weighed drug dosage and the prescription dosage. The dosage of each drug in the prescription should be accurate, and the dosage error of each drug should be controlled within ± 5%. Reweigh if necessary.

7.3.3 Recheck the medication problems such as antagonisms, mutual inhibitions of the medicine, contraindication in pregnancy and overdosage, and the correctness of dispensing toxic, anesthetic and expensive medicine.

7.3.4 Reviewing whether the drugs requiring special treatment such as decocted earlier, decocted later, wrap-boiling, melting, decocted separately, dissolving etc. are packaged separately and indicate the usage.

7.3.5 Recheck the quality of medicine, whether it is rotten due to insect bites or gets mouldy.

7.3.6 Recheck whether there is any problem of mistaken substitution, failing to distinguish the crude medicine from the processed one, or whether the medicine is mashed correctly.

7.3.7 Recheck the name, department, dispensing date and dosage of the tabs on the decocting canister and on the prescription for the resident prescription and the decoction medicine.

7.3.8 The medicine should not be packed until the reviewers checked and signed or sealed.

8 Dispensing Management of Special Decoction Pieces

It should comply with the relevant regulations of the health management departments of various countries and regions, and can also refer to Annex A for implementation.

Annex A
(Informative)
Dispensing Requirements of Special Chinese Medicines

A 1 Dispensing Management of Special Decoction Pieces

A 1.1 Dispensing and Management of Toxic Pieces for Medical Use

Toxic medicine cabinet should be set for the toxic medicines, the toxic medicines be kept by the certain stuffs in the certain account and be locked and tabbed in the special cabinet.

The doctor's signatures on the prescriptions are needed when medical units supplying and dispensing toxic medicines. During dispensing, the stuffs should be conscientious and have a sense of responsibility to account precisely and note the doctors' advices clearly, and the medicines should not be sent to the patients before the dispensing stuffs and reviewers with higher titles than pharmacist signed and sealed. The toxic medicines which are not noted with unprocessed should be dispensed with processed ones. Any questions about the prescriptions should be made clear to the doctors who prescripted before dispensing.

Specific account cards should be made for the toxic medicines, which should be reviewed every day and settled every month to ensure the consistency between accounts and goods. The registration book should be adopted to record the names, ages, workplaces, contact information of the patients, the names, amounts and expiring date of the medicines and the names of prescription doctors and dispensing stuffs.

The prescription should be used only once and the prescriptions and certificates should be kept for two years for future reference.

The toxic medicine variety scope, management, usages and dosages is recorded in SZJG 37.1-2011 *Specification of Prescription and Dispensing of Traditional Chinese Medicine—Part 1: Prescription of Traditional Chinese Medicine.*

A.1.2 Management and Dispensing of Anesthetic Chinese Decoction Pieces

The dispensing stuffs should dispense the anesthetic medicines with the specific prescriptions, and the pharmacist departments have the right to refuse dispensing to the illegal or improper prescriptions.

The prescriptions of dispensing anesthetic medicines should be recorded in the specific notebook, recording includes: date of dispensing, department, patient's name, medical record number, gender, age, diagnosis, the dosage of Pericarpium Papaveris, doctor's name, dispensing stuff and reviewer.

Shall not take medicine repeatedly with one prescription. After taking the medicine, the prescription shall be kept by the medical institution for 3 years for inspection.

A.1.3 Management and Dispensing of Expensive Chinese Decoction Pieces

The variety scope of expensive Chinese medicine is recorded in SZJG 37.1-2011 *Specification of Prescription and Dispensing of Traditional Chinese Medicine—Part 1: Prescription of Traditional Chinese Medicine*.

The first-class expensive Chinese medicine should be recorded into the account book, including: date, abstract of event, the amount of stock and selling, dispenser, reviewer. The prescription of dispensing should be set down one by one and be stored centralized, and the patient's name and the prescription number should be set down under the abstract of event.

Relevant management stuff should replenish medicines in time to ensure clinical medicines according to the consumption of outpatient medicines every day. The valuable medicines consumed on that day shall be registered and recorded in the account in time, and shall be consistent with the accounts receivable.

Expensive Chinese medicine should be checked regularly, outdated or moldy phenomenon should be prevented, and perishable medicine should be stored in locked freezers.

A. 2 List of Special Chinese Medicines

A. 2.1 Chinese Medicines with Incompatibility

Chinese medicines with incompatibility are shown in Table A.1.

Table A.1 Chinese Medicines with Incompatibility

Eighteen Clashes	Glycyrrhizae Radix et Rhizoma antagonises Kansui Radix , Euphorbiae Pekinensis Radix , Genkwa Flos and Sargassum. Aconite (Aconiti Radix , Aconiti Kusnezoffii Radix, Aconiti Lateralis Radix Preparata) antagonises Fritillaria Bulbus (Fritillariae Cirrhosae Bulbus, Fritillariae Thunbergii Bulbus , Fritillaria Ussuriensis Maxim, Fritillaria Pallidiflora Bulbus, Fritillaria Hupehensis Bulbus), Trichosanthis Fructus (Trichosanthis Fructus, Trichosanthis Semen, Trichosanthis Pericarpium, Trichosanthis Radix), Pinelliae Rhizoma, Ampelopsis Radix, Bletillae Rhizoma.Veratrum antagonises Ginseng Radix et Rhizoma, Salviae Miltiorrhizae Radix et Rhizoma, Glehniae Radix, Scrophulariae Radix, Sophorae Flavescentis Radix, Asari Radix et Rhizoma, Paeonia lactiflora Pall (Paeoniae Radix Alba and Paeoniae Radix Rubra)
Nineteen Incompatibilities	Sulfur restrains Natrii Sulfas. Hydrargyrum restrains white arsenic. Euphoriae Ebracteolata Radix restrains litharge.Crotonis Fructus restrains Pharbitidis Semen. Caryophylli Flos restrains Curcumae Radix. Aconiti Radix and Aconiti Kusnezoffii Radix restrain Rhino Horn. Natrii Sulfas restrains Sparganii Rhizoma. Cinnamomi Cortex restrains Halloysitum Rubrum. Ginseng Radix et Rhizoma restrains Trogopteri Faeces

A. 2.2 Chinese Medicines with Contraindications During Pregnancy

Chinese medicines with contraindications during pregnancy are shown in Table A.2.

Table A.2 Chinese Medicines with Contraindications During Pregnancy

Prohibited Drugs	Sparganii Rhizoma, Curcumae Rhizoma, Hirudo, Tabanus, Kansui Radix, Euphorbiae Pekinensis Radix, Genkwa Flos, Pharbitidis Semen, Crotonis Fructus, Euphorbiae Semen, Radix Phytolaccae, Calomelas, Mylabris, Realgar, Moschus, Gleditsiae Fructus Abnormalis, Leonuri Herba, Strychni Semen, Aconiti Lateralis Radix Preparata, Eupolyphaga Steleophaga, Cyathulae Radix, Natrii Sulfas Exsiccatus, Natrii Sulfas, Ferulae Resina, Rhododendron molle Flos, Scolopendra, etc.
Drugs Given Cautiously	Bufonis Venenum, Physochlainae Radix, Arisaematis Rhizoma Praeparatum, Toxicodendri Resina, Impatientis Semen, Sulfur, Acontiti Radix Cocta, Acontiti Kusnezoffii Radix Cocta, Typhonii Rhizoma, Aurantii Fructus Immaturus, Aurantii Fructus, Rhei Radix et Rhizoma, Sennae Folium, Cinnamomi Cortex, Campsis Flos, Momordicae Semen, Achyranthis Bidentatae Radix,Carthami Flos, Persicae Semen, Notoginseng Radix et Rhizoma, Pruni Semen, Polygoni Cuspidati Rhizoma et Radix, Selaginellae Herba, Selaginellae Herba, Echinopslatifolius Radix, Rhapontici Radix, Wenyujin Rhizoma Concisum, Croci Stigma, Manis Squama,Borneolum Syntheticum, Sappan Lignum, Tetrapanacis Medulla, Dichroae Radix, Pollen Typhae, Haematitum, Dianthi Herba, etc.

A. 2.3 Decoction Pieces Needed to be Decocted in Special Methods

Decoction pieces needed to be decocted in special methods are shown in Table A.3.

Tbale A.3 Decoction Pieces Needed to be Decocted in Special Methods

Decocted Earlier	Testudinis Carapax et Plastrum, Trionycis Carapax, Haematitum, Haliotidis Concha, Ostreae Concha, Draconis Os, Magnetitum, Fibrosum Gypsum, Fluoritum, Gypsum Rubrum, Pyritum, Gecko, Margaritifera Concha, Cervi Cornu Degelatinatum, Arcae Concha, Aconiti Radix Cocta, Aconiti Kusnezoffii Radix Cocta, Aconiti Lateralis Radix Preparata, Typhonii Rhizoma, Phytolaccae Radix, Arisaematis Rhizoma, Pinelliae Rhizoma, Dendrobii Caulis, etc.
Decocted Later	Menthae Haplocalycis Herba, Amomi Fructus,Ammomi Fructus Rotundus, Aquilariae Lignum Resinatum, Armeniacae Semen Amarum, Uncariae Ramulus cum Uncis, Rhei Radix et Rhizoma, Sennae Folium, Cynanchi Paniculati Radix et Rhizoma, Artemisiae Annuae Herba, Houttuyniae Herba,etc.
Wrap-boiling	Descurainiae Semen, Plantaginis Semen, Inulae Flos, Typhae Pollen, Liuyi powder, Daige powder, Yiyuan powder, Gecko, Indigo Naturalis, Lasiosphaera Calvatia, Talcum, Lygodii Spora, Catechu, etc.
Administered After Dissolved	Bovis Calculus, Notoginseng Radix, Margarita, Cinnabaris, Moschus, Ursi Fel, Calculus Equi, Calculus Macacae Mulattae, Saigae Tataricae Cornu, Aquilariae Resinatum Lignum, Amber, Eretmochelys Imbricata, Fritillariae Cirrhosae Bulbus, Fritillaria Hupehensis Bulbus, Omphalia, etc.
Melt	Asini Colla Corii, Cervi Corni Colla, Colla Carapax et Plastrum, Mel, Maltose, etc.
Decocted Separately	Ginseng Radix et Rhizoma, Gastrodiae Rhizoma, Cornu Saigae Tataricae, Panacis Quinquefolii Radix ,Croci Stigma, Cordyceps, Cornu Cervi Pantotrichum, etc.
Dissolving	Natrii Sulfas, Natrii Sulfas Exsiccatus, etc.

A. 2.4 Decoction Pieces Needed to be Pounded Temporarily

Decoction pieces needed to be pounded temporarily are shown in Table A.4.

TableA.4 Decoction Pieces Needed to be Pounded Temporarily

Fruits and Seeds	Caryophylli Flos, Canavaliae Semen, Jujubae Fructus, Toosendan Fructus, Schisandrae Chinensis Fructus, Arctii Fructus, Ginkgo Semen, Lablab Semen Album, Trichosanthis Fructus, Cassiae Semen, Galangae Fructus, Ammomi Fructus Rotundus, Sinapis Semen, Chebulae Fructus, Canarii Fructus, Pruni Semen, Quisqualis Fructus, Piperis Fructus, Piperis Longi Fructus, Alpiniae Katsumadai Semen, Tsaoko Fructus, Litchi Semen, Pharbitidis Semen, Amomi Fructus, Persicae Semen, Raphani Semen, Alpiniae Oxyphyllae Fructus, Akebiae Fructus, Gleditsiae Abnormalis Fructus, Sesami Semen Nigrum, Torreyae Semen, Ziziphi Spinosae Semen, Viticis Fructus, Prinsepiae Nux, Citri Reticulatae Semen, etc.
Roots and Stems	Cremastrae Pseudobulbus Pleiones Pseudobulbus, Fritillariae Ussuriensis Bulbus, Panacis Japonici Rhizoma, Physochlainae Radix, Panacis Majoris Rhizoma, Dryopteridis Crassirhizomatis Rhizoma,etc.
Minerals	Alumen, Pyritum, etc.
Animals	Hippocampus, Cervi Cornu Degelatinatum, Manis Squama, Trionycis Carapax, Testudinis Carapax et Plastrum, etc.
Others	Catechu, Cinnamomi Cortex, etc.